Cachet

Head Massage

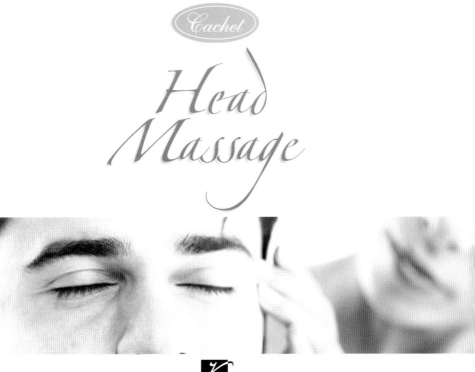

KUDOS

Published by Kudos, an imprint of Top That! Publishing plc.
Copyright © 2004 Top That! Publishing plc,
Tide Mill Way, Woodbridge, Suffolk, IP12 IAP, UK
www.kudosbooks.com
Kudos is a Trademark of Top That! Publishing plc

Contents

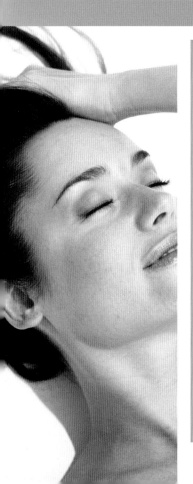

Introduction 3

Advantages of scalp massage 4

About your hair and scalp 6

Tips for hair and scalp health 8

Indian head massage......................................10

Step-by-step Indian head massage.................16

Different massage techniques 22

Give yourself a scalp massage 26

Massage a friend..28

Salon massage 32

Massage tools 34

Lotions and potions 36

Scalp massage oils 40

Scalp massage for health problems................42

General body massage...................................44

Conclusion 48

Introduction

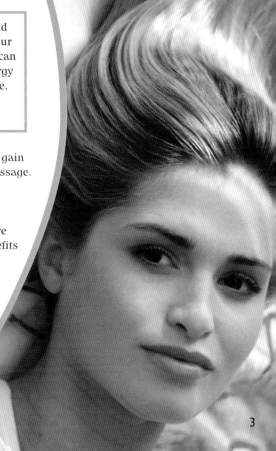

Massage – it's relaxing, sensual and health-giving. Unfortunately, with our busy all-day, on-the-go lifestyles, it can be difficult to find the time and energy to commit to a whole body massage, but a head massage can offer the perfect solution.

By concentrating on the head you can gain many of the benefits of an all-over massage. It's easier to find the time to fit in a head massage, and you can make it a regular part of your health and beauty routine. Not only will you become more relaxed, you will also gain all the benefits of a healthy scalp and hair.

There's plenty to learn about too. Whether you are planning to perform it on your own scalp, on a friend's, or just want to know about the basics before getting a professional head massage, the following pages will tell you all you need to know.

Advantages of scalp massage

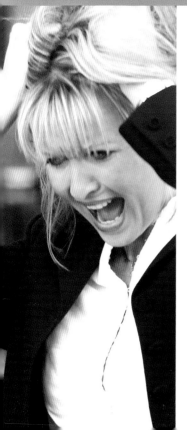

Many of us lead hectic lifestyles, balancing demanding work and family lives, which may leave us feeling stressed and tense.

Dealing with stress

Scalp massage is one of the best antidotes for dealing with stress, promoting feelings of wellbeing and encouraging the body's natural healing processes.

Where to get a scalp massage

Scalp massage can be done almost anywhere, whether you are at home, work, in a salon, school, hospital or clinic, and can be performed on anybody from babies to elderly people. It can be carried out while the recipient is fully clothed, saving time on getting dressed and undressed, and also benefiting those who are embarrassed to take their clothes off in front of other people.

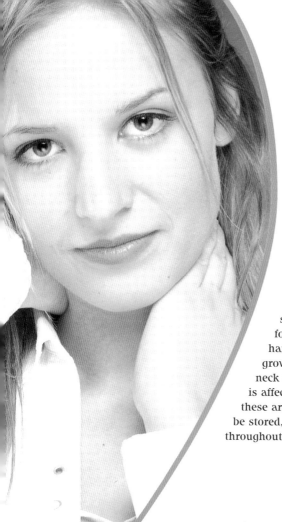

Treatments

Treatments can take place relatively quickly with only two willing participants needed. The use of oils is optional, so if for example you are at work, all you need to do after your massage is brush your hair back into place.

Health benefits

The benefits of scalp massage are many and varied. It offers relief from physical symptoms, such as headaches, migraines and stiff necks, and has calming, uplifting psychological benefits. Scalp massage also stimulates blood flow to hair follicles on the head, improving hair condition and encouraging hair growth. Although only the head and neck area is massaged, the entire body is affected. Once stress is released from these areas, common places for tension to be stored, energy can flow more freely throughout the whole body.

About your hair and scalp

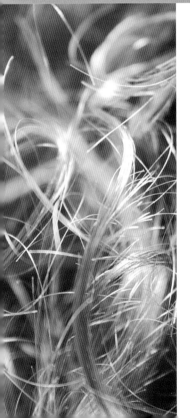

The skin on your scalp is thick and is usually covered in hair.

This skin is made up of three layers:

- a thin outer layer, or epidermis;
- a thick layer beneath this, called the dermis; and
- a deep layer of subcutaneous tissue containing fat.

Within the layers of skin are nerves, sweat and sebaceous glands. Nerves sense heat, cold, pain and touch. Sweat glands produce perspiration when you are hot, helping to regulate your body temperature. Sebaceous glands produce a lubricant, called sebum, which makes hair look shiny. Straight hair tends to look shinier because sebum from the sebaceous glands moves down the hair easily, while curlier hair may look duller as it is more difficult for sebum to move down the hair.

There are around five million hairs on your body, and about one million of these are on your head. Hair helps to keep you warm in cold weather, acts as a sensitive touch receptor and is an important factor in our gender and social identity.

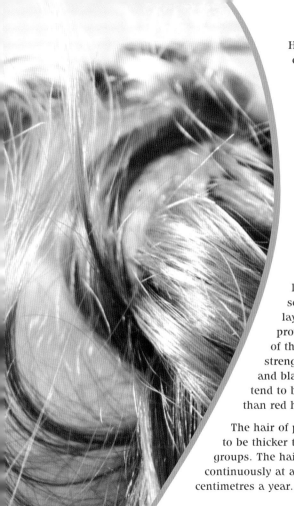

Hair follicles are situated in the epidermis and dermis layers of the skin. Hair grows out of the base of the hair follicle, which is a tube-shaped sheath surrounding the hair under the skin.

Small, sack-like glands, situated near the base of each follicle, release oils onto the hair follicles conditioning the hair and the surrounding skin. The shaft of each hair is made up of dead protein, called keratin. The outer layer of hair has scale-like layers and provides much of the hair's strength. Blonde and black hairs tend to be thinner than red hair.

The hair of people of African descent tends to be thicker than the hair of other ethnic groups. The hair on your head grows continuously at a rate of around ten centimetres a year.

7

Tips for hair and scalp health

A healthy scalp and hair is one of the most noticeable things about a person. Follow these ten terrific tips to keep your most visible assets in tiptop condition.

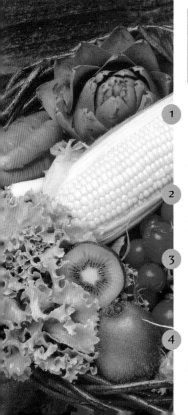

1. Lead a healthy lifestyle with a nutritious diet containing plenty of fresh fruit and vegetables, whilst minimising your intake of refined and processed foods. Avoid crash diets that can result in poor vitamin and mineral intake.

2. Excessive stress is not only harmful to your general wellbeing, but can also result in lank hair, or even loss of hair. Manage stress levels with relaxation techniques, exercise, fresh air and sleep.

3. Wash your hair regularly with a mild pH-balanced shampoo that is suitable for your hair type. Sweat and dirt can result in infected hair follicles and poor skin health. Rinsing after shampooing with cool water will give your hair shine.

4. Brush your hair at least twice a day to remove knots and impurities. Brushing stimulates the circulation to your scalp, increasing the amount of oxygen to the area and the release of natural oils.

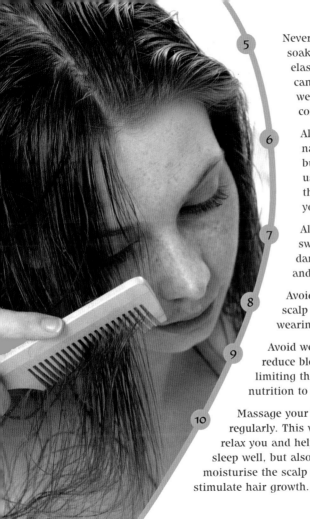

5   Never brush your hair when it is soaking wet as the hair is more elastic at this time and brushing can cause damage. Try combing wet hair with a wide-tooth comb to remove tangles.

6   Allow your hair to dry naturally whenever you can, but if you need to blow-dry it, use the lowest heat and keep the hair dryer as far from your scalp as possible.

7   Always wash your hair after swimming as chlorine has a damaging effect on the hair and scalp.

8   Avoid exposing your hair and scalp to the sun and wind by wearing a hat whenever possible.

9   Avoid wearing tight hats as they reduce blood circulation to the scalp, limiting the flow of oxygen and nutrition to the area.

10   Massage your head regularly. This will not only relax you and help you to sleep well, but also moisturise the scalp and stimulate hair growth.

Indian head massage

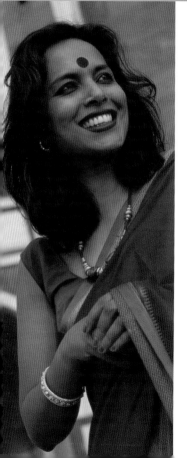

History

Indian head massage has been practised for over a thousand years in India. Also known as Champissage, it was developed by women to enhance the beauty and condition of their hair, encouraging the strong, glossy hair growth which Indian women are now famed for.

This form of massage is based on an ancient Indian system of medicine dating back over three thousand years. Known as 'Ayurveda', which translated means 'knowledge of life', this traditional art form is based on the holistic approach to living which involves balancing the body, mind and soul to promote health and happiness.

Development

Narendra Metha, a blind man from India, developed Indian head massage into a formal therapy. He trained as a physiotherapist in England in the 1970s, and then returned to India to study Champissage. He added his knowledge of shiatsu and acupuncture and extended the massage to include the face, neck and shoulders – areas that tend to become very tense.

Indian head massage is increasingly recognised in the West as having excellent therapeutic benefits.

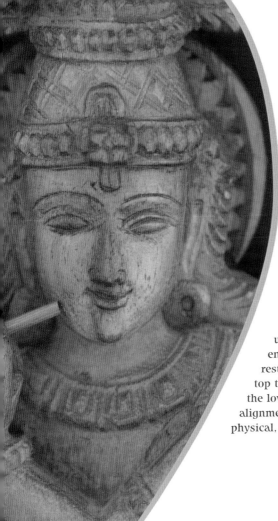

Theory

It is thought that the body has spinning centres of energy, called 'chakras', which should be in harmony and alignment to maintain physical, mental and emotional balance. The aim of an Indian head massage is to balance the chakras.

What are chakras?

Indian head massage works on the three higher chakras – Visuddha (the throat), Ajna (the brow) and Sahasrara (the crown). The chakras can be blocked or damaged by emotional upset, anxiety or stress. When the chakras are unblocked and free from negative energy, balance and harmony are restored. It is believed that when the top three chakras are balanced, the lower chakras will vibrate into alignment, resulting in improved physical, mental and spiritual health.

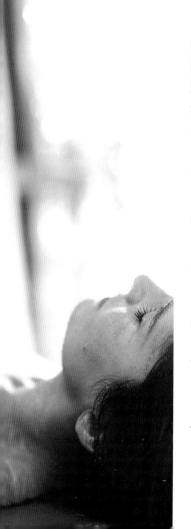

Benefits of Indian head massage

Indian head massage is a gentle and naturally therapeutic treatment which works on areas of the body affected by physical and emotional stress. The benefits include:

- a calming, uplifting and relaxing effect through the release of endorphins (the 'feel-good' chemicals);

- stimulated circulation and increased blood flow to the brain, resulting in increased oxygen and glucose which improves memory and concentration;

- the relaxation of stiff and tight muscles through the breakdown of tension knots, eliminating toxic products and increasing the mobility of joints;

- increased lymphatic drainage which helps to remove toxins and boosts the body's immune system, helping it to fight infections;

- the reduction of the frequency of headaches, migraine and eye strain through the relief of tension;

- improved skin condition and hair growth through the stimulation of sweat and sebaceous glands, increasing blood flow to the scalp and eliminating waste products; and

- possible relief from insomnia and depression through the calming, soothing and uplifting effects of massage.

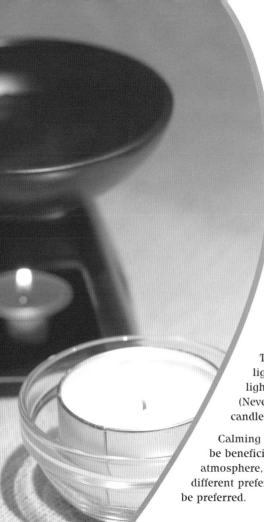

Preparing for an Indian head massage

Choose a time and place when you are unlikely to be interrupted. Being disturbed during a massage can result in feelings of tension, reducing the effects of the massage. Turn on the answerphone and switch off your mobile phone.

Make sure the room is warm and well ventilated, but not draughty.

Ensure you have everything to hand before you start, such as towels, oils and pillows or cushions.

Turn down any bright lights and, if possible, light a few candles. (Never leave burning candles unattended).

Calming background music can be beneficial in creating a tranquil atmosphere, though each person has different preferences and silence may be preferred.

13

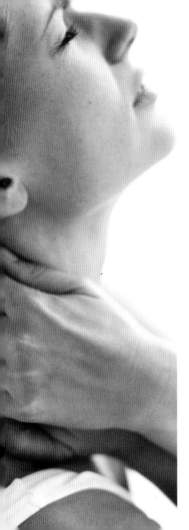

Warning signs

Although Indian head massage is a gentle and, in most cases, a very safe therapy, there are a few instances when it is not suitable. If there are any doubts as to the health or wellbeing of the recipient, a medical practitioner should be consulted before commencing with any massage. The recipient's age and individual needs should be taken into consideration, and the pressure moderated accordingly.

If the recipient has any of the following conditions, Indian head massage should not be carried out:

- any skin condition, swelling, inflammation or bruising in the area to be massaged;

- recent injury or surgery to the head, neck or shoulders;

- fever, high temperature or infections such as flu, a cough, cold or chest infection;

- very high, or low, blood pressure;

- any serious medical condition whilst undergoing treatment; or

- if the recipient has a known blood clot. This could become dislodged by the massage, blocking a blood vessel.

Allow seven to ten days between treatments to allow toxins released by the previous treatment to be eliminated.

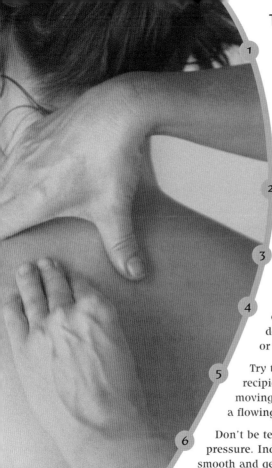

Top tips for massage

1. Make sure that the recipient is sitting comfortably, with their legs uncrossed and their feet placed flat on the ground. Removing their shoes will help the recipient feel more relaxed. A pillow placed on their lap will provide a comfortable place to rest their hands.

2. Encourage them to tell you if they feel uncomfortable, or if they experience any pain or discomfort.

3. Talk only when necessary as this can be distracting and will disrupt the flow of the massage.

4. Be sure that your posture is correct whilst massaging so you don't cause yourself any strain or discomfort.

5. Try to keep your hands on the recipient throughout the massage, moving from one stroke to the other in a flowing movement.

6. Don't be tempted to apply too much pressure. Indian head massage should be smooth and gentle.

Step-by-step Indian head massage

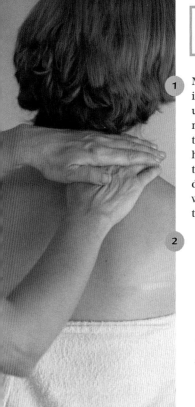

It's time to get hands on, so follow the steps below for the perfect massage technique.

1 Make sure the recipient is sitting comfortably; use pillows or cushions if necessary. Stand behind the recipient and rest your hands lightly on their head, then ask them to take some deep breaths, concentrating while exhaling to reduce any tension in the body.

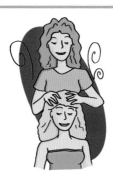

2 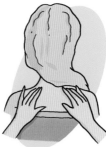 If you are using oil, rub a small amount into the palm of your hands to warm it, then position your hands on either side of the spine with your fingers on the shoulders. Use your palms to make large, circular stroking movements across the shoulders and upper back.

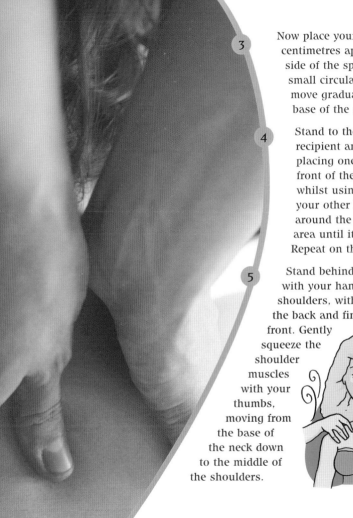

3 Now place your thumbs a few centimetres apart on either side of the spine, and, using small circular movements, move gradually up to the base of the neck.

4 Stand to the side of the recipient and reach across, placing one hand on the front of their shoulder, whilst using the palm of your other hand to rub around the shoulder blade area until it feels warm. Repeat on the other side.

5 Stand behind the recipient with your hands on their shoulders, with your thumbs to the back and fingers to the front. Gently squeeze the shoulder muscles with your thumbs, moving from the base of the neck down to the middle of the shoulders.

17

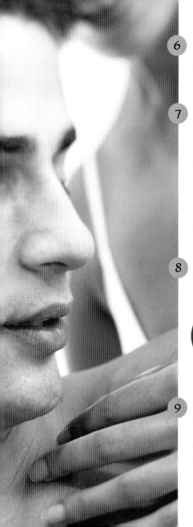

6 Now place both fingers and thumbs over the shoulders, press the base of your palms into the back and roll the muscles over the top of the shoulder blades.

7 Stand behind the recipient with your forearms resting on their shoulders, your fists loosely clenched and facing upwards. Glide your forearms across from the neck, working out towards the top of the arms, while at the same time rotating your forearms so that your fists are facing downwards. Repeat five times.

8 Stand to the side of the recipient and place one hand at the back, and one hand at the front of the upper arm. Squeeze the arm gently and then release, moving slowly down the arm towards the elbow. Keeping your hands in contact with the recipient, slide them back up the arm and repeat the action. Repeat on the other arm.

9 Standing to the side of the recipient, place one hand on the shoulder and the other supporting their elbow. Rotate the shoulder around clockwise, then anticlockwise, three times in each direction. Repeat on the other shoulder.

10 Stand to the side of the recipient with one hand on the back of their neck and one on their forehead. Very gently rotate the head clockwise and then anticlockwise, keeping the movement very slow. Repeat three times in each direction.

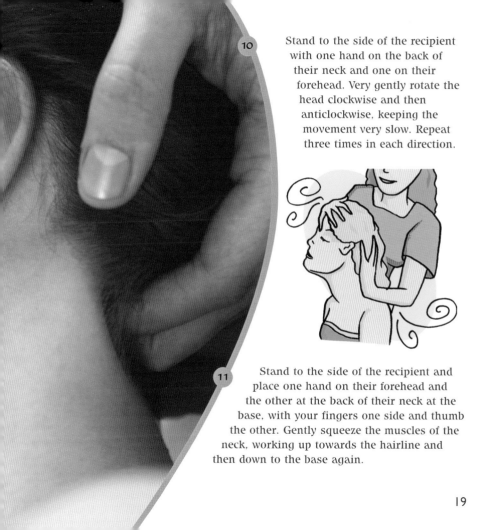

11 Stand to the side of the recipient and place one hand on their forehead and the other at the back of their neck at the base, with your fingers one side and thumb the other. Gently squeeze the muscles of the neck, working up towards the hairline and then down to the base again.

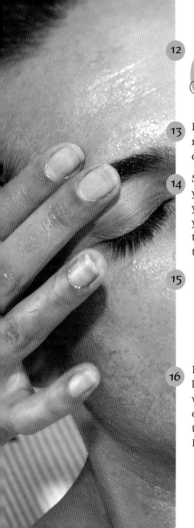

12 Stand at the back of the recipient and pick up small amounts of hair in each hand, tugging gently. Work around the whole head, so that all the hair is picked up.

13 Hold your hands above the recipient's head, and gently tap all over their scalp with your fingertips.

14 Stand behind the recipient and place your hands on their forehead with your fingers overlapping and facing each other. Sweep your hands outwards towards the temples, then bring them back into the original position without lifting them off the face. Repeat four to five times.

15 Stand still behind the recipient, placing your hands on their cheeks with your fingers pointing towards their nose. Stroke gently, but firmly, outwards towards their ears. Repeat four to five times.

16 In the same position, place both your hands on the chin with your fingers facing each other. Stroke outwards along the jaw bone towards the ears. Repeat no more than five times.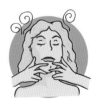

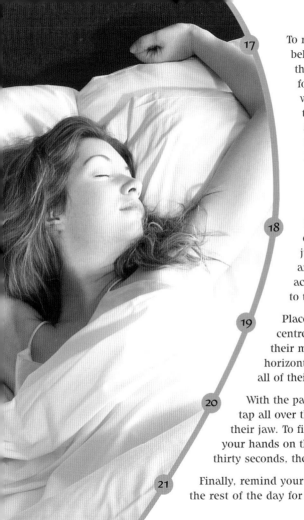

17 To relieve pressure points, stand behind the recipient with your thumbs in the centre of their forehead below their hairline, with your fingers resting on their cheeks. Gently press and release, with your thumbs working outwards in horizontal lines. Bring your thumbs back to the centre and repeat down the forehead to the eyebrows.

18 Now place your forefingers on the bridge of their nose just below their eyes. Press and release in horizontal lines across their cheekbones down to their mouth.

19 Place your forefingers on the centre of their chin just below their mouth. Press and release in horizontal rows, as above, covering all of their chin.

20 With the pads of your forefingers gently tap all over their face, including under their jaw. To finish the massage, gently rest your hands on the recipient's head for about thirty seconds, then gradually lift your hands.

21 Finally, remind your recipient to take it easy for the rest of the day for maximum benefit.

21

Different massage techniques

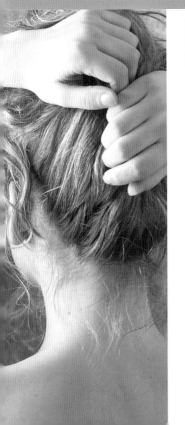

There are many different techniques used to massage the scalp and head. Some of them are easy to learn and can be practised at home, while others should only be performed by a qualified therapist.

Hair-pulling massage

This is a very simple technique to learn and easy to perform on yourself. This form of massage helps relieve tension in the muscles that are attached to your hair, increasing the flow of blood to the brain and leaving you calm, but alert.

As much of your nervous system is in your brain, hair-pulling massage is very effective in stimulating the nerve pathways and activating little-used cells. Due to the release of endorphins, anxiety levels are reduced and feelings of calm and wellbeing are induced. It can be helpful in treating headaches, migraines, sinus problems, stress and tension, aches and stiffness in the body.

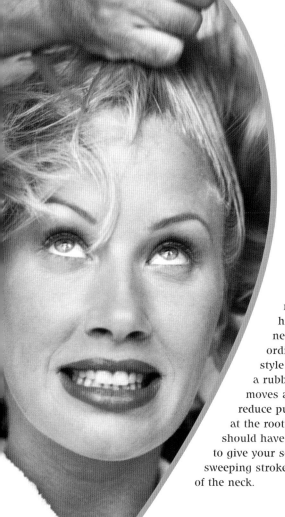

Take a small section of hair between the thumb and forefinger and gently tug the hair, sliding your fingers from the scalp to the end of the hair. Start at the front of your hair and work your way to the back of your head, circling round to the crown. Continue until all the hair on your head has been tugged. Do not pull so hard that hair comes out. The pressure should feel comfortable, not painful.

Hairbrush massage

One of the easiest ways to massage your scalp is by using a hairbrush. No special equipment is needed, although an ordinary, flat paddle-style brush with a rubber base that moves a little will reduce pulling your hair at the roots. The brush should have dense bristles to give your scalp a good workout. Use long, sweeping strokes from the forehead to the nape of the neck.

23

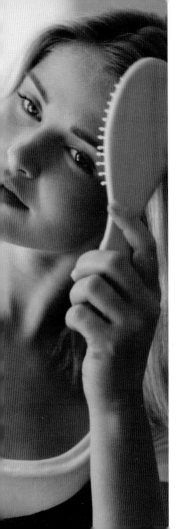

Scalp rapping

Based on an Indonesian massage technique, this is designed to increase the circulation to the scalp and promote healthy hair growth.

Stand with your feet apart and breathe deeply. Keep your legs straight and lean forward from the waist, bringing your head down to just below your waist. Rap your scalp with your knuckles, tapping gently for about thirty seconds. Slowly come back up to a standing position and repeat the process.

Yoga headstand

For those of you who are brave enough, this is very beneficial for increasing the blood supply to the brain and scalp, and improving the health of your hair. Other benefits can include improved memory, fewer headaches, relief from asthma and better sleep patterns. If you are a novice headstander, start in a corner which will provide some support if you start to fall, or ask someone to help you.

You will need some padding for your head, such as a yoga mat, foam pad or folded blanket, but not a pillow as it is too soft. If you are worried about falling, place a pillow behind your head.

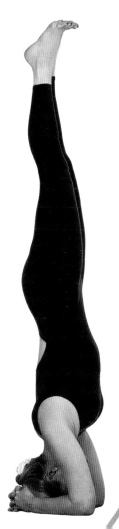

Kneel down on the floor with your arms in front of you and your fingers interlocked, placing them close to the corner of the wall.

Place your head against the palms of your hands and straighten your legs. Your body should not experience any discomfort, so don't force any position.

Lift one leg up and place it against the wall. Then kick the other leg up and place it next to the first.

Stay in this position for fifteen to twenty seconds, slowly increasing the time to around three minutes as you become more used to the position.

To come down from a headstand simply lower one leg at a time, keeping your movements as smooth as possible.

With practice your confidence and balance will improve and you will find it becomes easier to get in and out of this position.

Give yourself a scalp massage

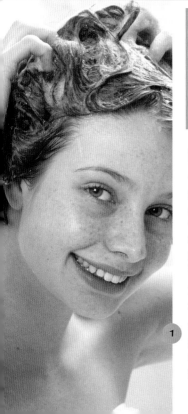

Scalp massage is not only relaxing and invigorating, it can also benefit your hair's health. It stimulates circulation, increasing oxygen and nutrient supplies to your scalp and hair follicles. This will improve the condition of your scalp and hair, promote hair growth, and can even help prevent hair loss.

In the shower

You can give yourself a scalp massage at any time and in any place, but the easiest way to increase the circulation to your scalp is to massage your head when you are shampooing your hair. Use your fingertips or knuckles, depending on the pressure that you prefer, and move over the scalp, temples and the back of your head using circular movements.

Follow these steps to give yourself a relaxing scalp massage, whether in or out of the shower.

1 Using the pads of your index and middle fingers, make small circles all over your head. Start at the temples and work around until you have covered all of your head.

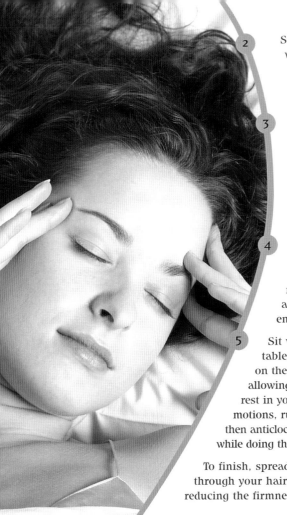

2 Stroke your scalp firmly, working in the direction of the hair growth, running your fingers through your hair at the end of each stroke.

3 Out of the shower, when the hair is dry, take small sections of hair and tug firmly but gently (this should not hurt, nor should hair be pulled out), working over the whole of the head.

4 Place your forefingers on either side of your temples and, using circular motions, rub first clockwise, then anticlockwise, covering the entire temple area.

5 Sit with your elbows resting on a table. Place the heel of your hand on the space between your eyebrows, allowing the weight of your head to rest in your hand. Using circular motions, rub the spot first clockwise, then anticlockwise. Remember to sit upright while doing this, with your spine straight.

To finish, spread your fingers and run them through your hair. Start quite firmly, gradually reducing the firmness.

Massage a friend

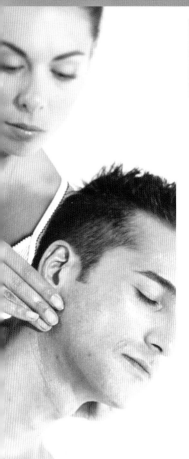

Why not give a friend a real treat and give them a head and neck massage? Follow these easy tips to provide a pampering experience your friend will never forget.

Set the mood

Make sure you have enough time to complete the massage and won't be interrupted. Turn off mobile phones and hang a 'do not disturb sign' on the door! Make sure the room to be used is warm and draught free. Relaxing music, such as classical or 'mood' pieces, will create a calming atmosphere. Turn off harsh lighting, and use lamps or candlelight (never leave burning candles unattended). An oil burner with a suitable essential oil, diluted in water, can provide a lovely, relaxing scent in the room.

Get ready

Wear loose, comfortable clothing and remove any rings or watches that may scratch. Have everything you need close to hand. Decide whether your friend will be sitting or lying down and use pillows to make them comfortable.

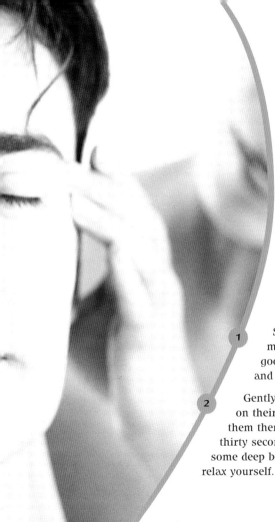

Discuss with your friend whether they have any allergies or sensitivities, and decide whether you will give a 'dry' massage or one using oils.

During a massage, be aware of your friend's body language and their rate and depth of breathing. Watch out for any stiffening of muscles, sharp intakes of breath, or hunching of the shoulders which are all indications of pain or discomfort. Comb their hair before you start to remove any tangles.

The massage

1 Stand squarely behind your friend, making sure that your posture is good. Shake your hands to relax them and to release any tension.

2 Gently place your hands on their head, resting them there for around thirty seconds. Take some deep breaths to relax yourself.

29

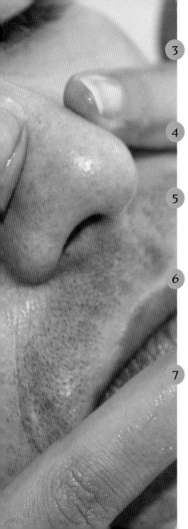

3 Hold your hands on either side of their head. With the heels of your hands, make firm, gentle circles over the entire scalp.

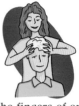

4 Support their head by placing the fingers of one hand on their forehead. With the palm of the other hand, rub all over their head, using brisk movements. Start from the base of their head and work up to the crown.

5 Spread your fingers and thumbs out on their head, and make small, circular movements over the scalp, using only the pads of your fingers, as though you were shampooing their hair. Massage along the hairline and around the ears and back of the neck.

6 Pick up small amounts of hair between your thumb and forefinger, lifting the hair up and giving it a gentle tug as you do so. Work over the entire head, including all the hair.

7 Place your hands on either side of their head with your fingers pointing towards their face. Stroke the head starting at the top using your hands alternately. Start one hand as the other is finishing its stroke so that there is continuous movement.

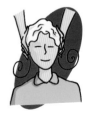

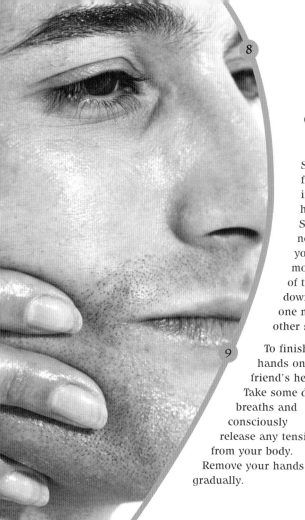

8

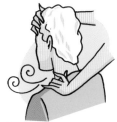

Stand to one side of your friend. Support their head in one hand by placing a hand on the forehead. Stroke down the side of the neck furthest away from you in a sweeping movement. Start at the top of their neck and continue down to their shoulders in one movement. Repeat on the other side.

9

To finish off, gently rest your hands on your friend's head. Take some deep breaths and consciously release any tension from your body. Remove your hands gradually.

Salon massage

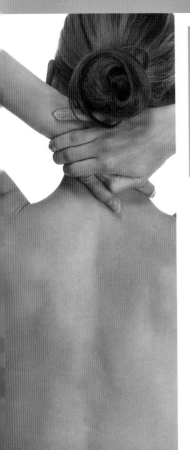

There are many different salon treatments available. A visit to a salon should be a relaxing and rejuvenating experience. Trained staff can give you a professional massage, and provide specialised therapy aimed at treating and nurturing the mind, body and spirit, as well as attending to specific problem areas. Cranial sacral and Shirodhara are just two of the treatments available at many salons.

Cranial sacral therapy

This therapy is used to release tension and energy blocks from the head to the bottom of the spine, the sacrum. Cerebrospinal fluid bathes the brain and spinal cord and one of its functions is to cushion them from injury. Messages from the brain travel down the spinal cord and are then sent to all parts of the body. It is believed that any blockage in the flow of cerebrospinal fluid can cause related problems in other parts of the body.

Manipulating the bones of the head, spine and sacrum by gentle massage can release blockages and improve the flow of cerebrospinal fluid.

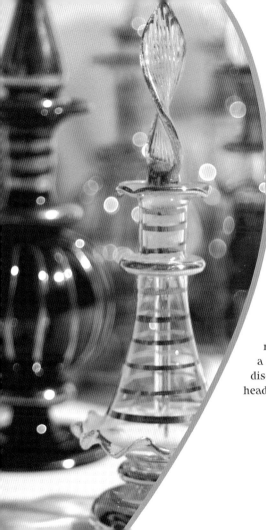

Shirodhara

Shirodhara is an Ayurvedic treatment. The word 'shirodhara' is a combination of two Sanskrit words – 'shiro', meaning head and 'dhara', meaning flow. It is a purifying and rejuvenating therapy designed to eliminate toxins from the body and relieve stress and mental exhaustion.

During the therapy warm oil is poured, or dripped, onto the forehead for around twenty to thirty minutes. This is usually followed by a scalp massage.

Shirodhara is a very relaxing therapy, aimed at eliminating toxins, while nourishing and replenishing the body. It can be a useful therapy for a variety of disorders such as stress, insomnia, headaches, rheumatism and asthma.

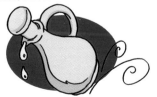

Massage tools

There are many different scalp massage tools on the market, with some of them looking as though they come from outer space. If you fancy using a tool to aid your own massage technique, have a look to see what is available.

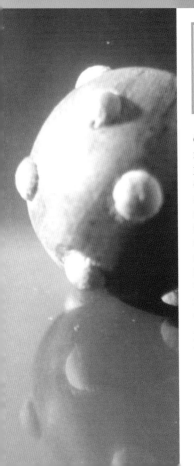

One of the strangest looking massage tools has long prongs which are designed to massage the acupressure points on the scalp. These prongs stimulate the nerve endings, resulting in a tingling sensation from head to toe. This tool can either be used manually, or motorised. Care needs to be taken to avoid the eyes, and it is not recommended for people with heart conditions or pacemakers.

Spiky rubber or wooden balls can be used to massage not only the scalp, but the whole body, too.

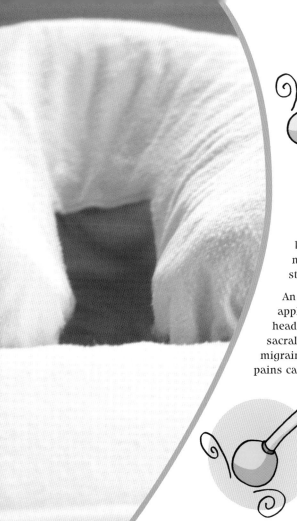

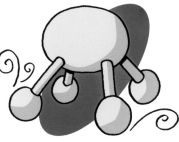

A simple and effective massage tool is one with round wooden balls which can be used to massage the scalp or any other part of the body. This helps relieve muscular tension and stimulates the circulation.

An ergonomically-designed pillow applies pressure to the back of the head, and is an aid to cranial sacral therapy. Headaches, migraines and general aches and pains can be relieved.

Rubber balls on the end of flexible metal rods are great for all-over massage and are said to relieve tension headaches.

Lotions and potions

There is a bewildering amount of products available in the hair care market. Here are a few alternatives for you to try. All of them use ingredients that are cheap and easy to find, as well as being good for your scalp.

The skin is the largest organ of the body, and the scalp is part of this. Like the rest of your skin, your scalp can be dry, normal, or oily. This, in turn, has an effect on your hair. If your skin is dry, your scalp is probably dry too, and likewise if it is oily.

There are many products to choose from that will keep your scalp and hair in great condition. Always choose products designed for your particular hair or skin type. If you have oily hair or skin, for example, choose products that are specifically for this problem. Products containing natural ingredients are usually milder and more gentle on your skin.

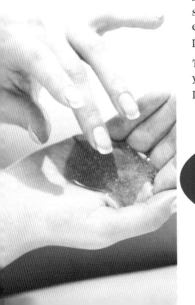

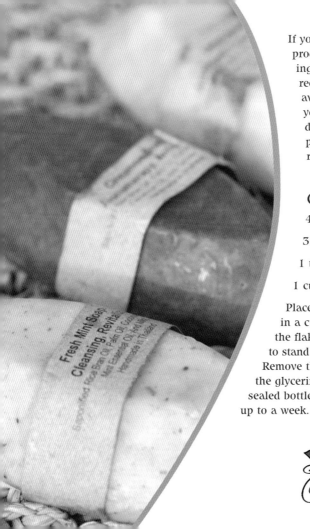

If you prefer to make your own products from all-natural ingredients, here are a few recipes to try. Remember to avoid any products to which you have an allergy, and discontinue using any products to which your skin reacts adversely.

Chamomile shampoo

4 chamomile tea bags

3 tablespoons pure soap flakes

1 tablespoon glycerine

1 cup of boiled water

Place the tea bags and soap flakes in a cup of boiled water. Stir until the flakes have dissolved. Allow to stand for fifteen to twenty minutes. Remove the bags and discard. Add the glycerine and stir well. Keep in a sealed bottle in a cool, dark place, for up to a week.

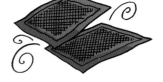

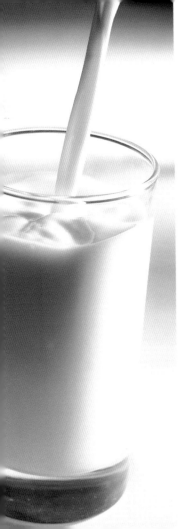

Hair and scalp conditioner

This conditioner helps to remove impurities from the pores on the scalp, allowing nutrients to reach the hair.

200 ml skimmed milk

1 egg yolk

1 tablespoon wheat germ

1 teaspoon olive oil

Blend all ingredients together. Massage the mixture into your scalp. Leave in for ten minutes then rinse with warm water. Shampoo and condition your hair as normal.

Hot oil treatment

This treatment can be used to treat dry hair, dandruff and split ends.

120 ml boiling water

120 ml olive oil

Mix the oil and water together, then leave the mixture to cool until it is hand hot, but not hot enough to burn. Place the mixture in a glass bottle or jar. Shake very well. Massage into your hair, wrap your hair in a towel and leave it for twenty minutes. Shampoo with your regular product and rinse.

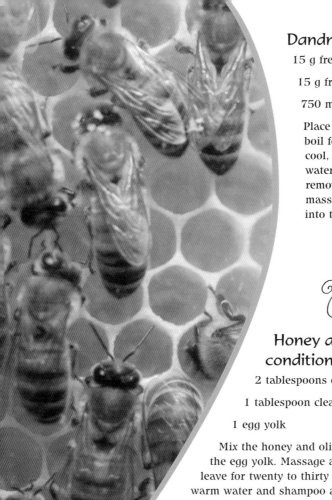

Dandruff treatment

15 g fresh sage leaves

15 g fresh rosemary leaves

750 ml water

Place herbs into the water and boil for five minutes. Allow to cool, leaving the leaves in the water. When the water is cool, remove the leaves and massage the infused water into the scalp. Do not rinse.

Honey and egg conditioner

2 tablespoons olive oil

1 tablespoon clear honey

1 egg yolk

Mix the honey and olive oil together. Beat in the egg yolk. Massage all over the hair and leave for twenty to thirty minutes. Rinse with warm water and shampoo as normal.

Scalp massage oils

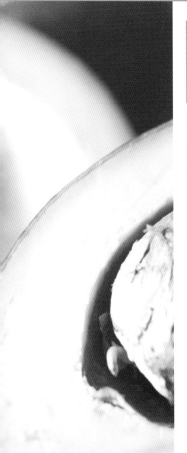

As essential oils are absorbed deeply into the skin, they can have powerful effects. They aid skin regeneration, fight infections and alleviate stress. Mental and emotion wellbeing also benefit.

> ⚠ **WARNING**
>
> Essential oils enter the bloodstream through the skin. NEVER apply them directly to your skin as they can be extremely potent. Dilute in a carrier oil and ALWAYS do a patch test first.
>
> Patch test: Mix one drop of the essential oil into a teaspoon of carrier oil. Rub a little of the mixture on the inside of your wrist. Leave uncovered and unwashed for 24 hours. If you suffer no redness or itching the oil is safe to use in a diluted form.

The following base oils are suitable to use on the scalp. Essential oils can then be added to treat specific problems, essential oils should always be diluted with a carrier oil before use on the skin.

- olive oil – healing qualities and skin conditioner.

- jojoba oil – supports longevity and has similar qualities to the body's own natural oil, sebum.

- grapeseed oil – regenerative and moisturising.

- avocado oil – aids skin elasticity and regeneration, moisturises.

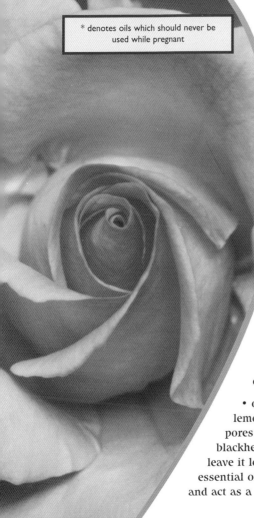

If you are pregnant, breast-feeding or suffer from any medical condition, consult your doctor, or a qualified aromatherapist, before using any essential oils.

Some oils only last a few weeks, such as lemon, so note the date on the bottle or label. The following essential oils can be blended with a base oil for massaging and treating your hair and scalp:

• all types: lavender, rose, geranium, ylang ylang and chamomile. These are very gentle and safe and suitable for use on all skin and hair types

• dry: *rosemary, *sage, *cedarwood, sandalwood and frankincense. These oils encourage the production of the body's natural oils in the skin and scalp.

• oily: *clary sage, *basil, lemon, lemongrass and *myrtle. Oil can clog the pores in the skin leading to pimples and blackheads. Excessive oil on the hair can leave it looking dull and lifeless. These essential oils help reduce the production of oil and act as a mild antiseptic to treat infection.

Scalp massage for health problems

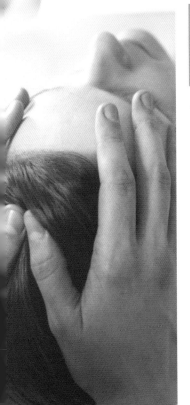

Massage and similar therapies are increasingly being used to enhance and complement traditional treatments such as surgery, radiotherapy and chemotherapy, and to boost the immune system.

Proven to help

Massage can be used hand-in-hand with conventional therapy in many areas of medicine including cancer care, geriatrics, maternity and neonatal care. It has been proven to decrease blood pressure, heart rate and respiratory rate. It can also provide pain relief through the release of endorphins, which are the body's natural pain killers. Blood flow to vital organs is increased and the immune system bolstered.

Scalp massage alleviates stress and the build-up of emotional and physical tension, helping the body to function more effectively. If stress accumulates with no release it can lead to physical and emotional ill-health, such as stomach ulcers, headaches, migraine, high blood pressure and depression.

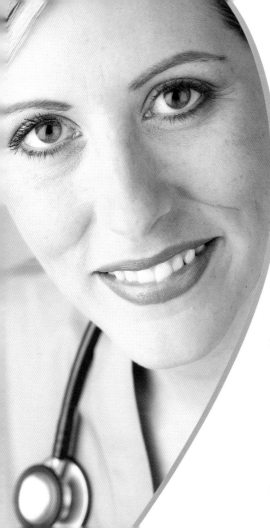

Medical advice

Disease and ill health can cause stress and anxiety, which scalp massage helps to alleviate. However, as with all treatments that have an impact on your health, if you are considering using head massage as part of a treatment regime for a serious or extensive problem, you should certainly seek professional advice from your GP or other doctor before starting.

In any case or situation, you should be wary of anyone that insists that head, or any other massage, will take the place of medication that you have been prescribed.

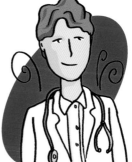

General body massage

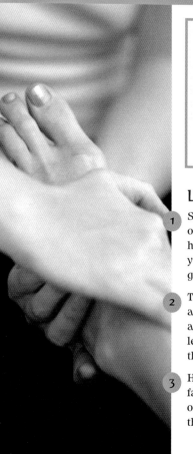

If you've enjoyed scalp massage, why not try a full body massage? Use a carrier oil with or without essential oils, depending on the recipient's preference and skin tolerance (see warning on page 40). Prepare for the massage as you would for an Indian head massage, placing a thick layer of blankets or towels on the floor for the recipient to lie on. Do not massage anybody with a medical problem or illness without consulting a doctor first.

Legs and feet

1. Start at the front of the body with the recipient lying on their back. Kneel to one side of their feet with your hands crossed over the left ankle. Slide the palms of your hands up the leg to the thigh, using firm but gentle pressure.

2. Turn your hands so that your fingers face forwards, and bring them down the sides of the left leg to the ankle. Finish by running one hand over the top of the left foot and the other on the sole of the foot. Repeat the steps 1 and 2 twice more.

3. Hold your hands over the left thigh with your palms facing each other. Flick your hands from the wrists, one after the other, striking the thigh with the edge of the hand, using light and bouncy movements.

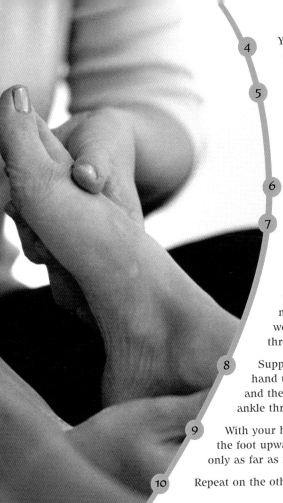

4. You can do this movement on the calf muscle too, but avoid the bony area at the front of the leg.

5. Cup your hands onto the left thigh using quick movements. You should hear a loud cupping sound, but it should not be uncomfortable for the recipient.

6. Stroke the leg again, as in the first two steps.

7. Support the left foot in your hands, with your fingers underneath the foot and thumbs on top. Work your thumb in the areas between the tendons, using small circular movements. Start at the toes and work towards the ankle. Repeat three times in each space.

8. Support the foot again by placing one hand under the leg just above the ankle and the other on the toes. Rotate the ankle three times in each direction.

9. With your hands in the same position, flex the foot upwards and then stretch it down. Go only as far as is comfortable for the recipient.

10. Repeat on the other leg.

45

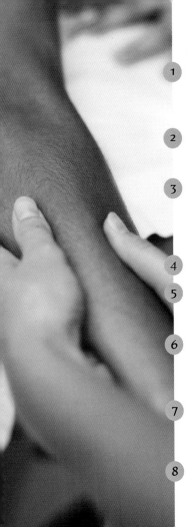

Arms and hands

1. Kneel next to the right side of the recipient. Support their right wrist in one hand, using the other to sweep up the arm, starting at the wrist. Continue round the right shoulder and down again. Repeat three times.

2. Place the recipient's right hand on your shoulder for support. Knead their upper arm by picking up and squeezing the muscles, beginning at the elbow.

3. Lower the arm, with the recipient's elbow on the towel. Support the arm with one hand, using the other to knead the inside of the arm. Move from the wrist to the elbow. Slide your hands back down to the wrist and repeat three times.

4. Repeat the first stroke again.

5. Support the recipient's right hand in your own. Stroke between the tendons of the hand as you did on the foot, working from the knuckles to the wrist.

6. Using your thumb, press gently in a circular motion round the joints of each of the fingers, beginning at the tip. Then gently rotate each finger in turn, both clockwise and anticlockwise.

7. Bend their arm up at the elbow, supporting it with one hand. Hold their hand in yours, locking fingers together. Rotate the hand from the wrist in both directions.

8. Repeat on the left arm.

Back and shoulders

1. Kneel to either one side of the recipient, or straddle them with a leg either side of their buttocks, not putting any of your weight on their back. Never massage on the spine.

2. Start at the lower back, with your hands on either side of the spine. Pressing firmly, slide your hands up the back in one continuous movement. Sweep your hands around the shoulders and bring your hands down the sides of the body and back to the original position. Repeat three times.

3. Place your hands on either side of the spine, level with the shoulder blades. Make small circles with your thumbs, working up to the base of the neck.

4. Kneeling on one side of the recipient, knead their side furthest away from you, picking up and releasing the muscles alternately with each hand. Work from the waist to the shoulders. Repeat on the other side.

5. Repeat the first stroke again.

Conclusion

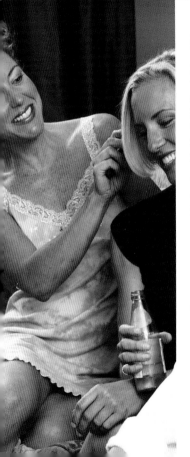

Mini massage

Many people say that the most enjoyable part of a visit to the hairdresser is having their hair washed by someone else. Part of this enjoyment comes from letting another person take the strain for a short while, part from the close physical contact, and part from the actual rhythm of the washing. A good head massage is just like this… only much, much better.

While some complementary and 'new age' therapies offer little or no proven benefits, a head massage is a low-key but guaranteed stress-busting treat.

Make new friends

Once you have absorbed the basics of how to give a good head massage you may soon find that friends you didn't even know you had are queuing up for a sample of your services. Just remember to leave some time for yourself or you will be back to square one in the stress stakes.

So, it's time to put the book down and head off for your first massage.